Contents

Chapter 1

Introduction

The author of this writing, aims to look at Corporate Social Responsibility – CSR- from a new perspective. For that he goes through worldview and teaching of an ancient philosopher and teacher named "Zarathushtra". These teachings and worldview are reflected from Zarathushtra's thought provoking book called "The Gathas".

The idea of working on this topic was shaping in the author's mind, more strongly when he was studying at the third semester of Bachelor of Hospitality Management. In that period, he had to study a study unit named "Corporate Social Responsibility". But on the other hand, simultaneously, he had started to study and learn about Zoroastrianism and Zarathushtra's philosophy by himself out of school. The more he learned about Zoroastrianism and CSR separately, the more he was finding similarities among them.

Therefore, he was inspired to pay more attention to these two topics, as well as applying Zarathushtra's philosophy in the organizational management field. This was almost the beginning point of a process, which eventually reached to publish of this book. To obtain the objectives of this writing, the author has studied CSR; and at the same time he continued studying Zarathushtra's philosophy related to it.

Nowadays, in managerial and organizational field, CSR is one of the very considerable topics. Planet earth has been suffering a lot since the industrial revolution, due to human activities against the nature. These days, many universities in different countries pay more attention to CSR, due to an understanding of its importance. On the other hand, there is much ancient wisdom unknown to many people in different fields, especially related to CSR. By taking all mentioned points into account, the writer of this material found it useful to work with the Gathas' wisdom, which can be beneficial for the future of CSR's filed as well as managerial filed.

In short, CSR aims for awakening us to be more caring and responsible about our human activities. On the other hand, Zarathushtra taught us for transferring human to become more caring, in order to make the world constantly happier, more comfortable, and more developing place. Therefore, there are many similar points of view in the field of CSR and the Gathas. And by knowing this fact, out of all similarities; the author has collected three common points of view in this writing.

As a matter of the fact that both CSR and Zarathustra's philosophy include a wide variety of aspects, therefore, only three of them will be taken into consideration in this writing. These are included of Environmental, Social, and Organizational aspects. The process of this work was included of studying CSR, the Gathas, and writings of other experts in Zoroastrianism field.

In the following chapters, there will be a glance at Zarathushtra's life, his philosophy and worldview, and CSR. Environmental, social, and organizational aspects in both, teaching of Zarathustra and CSR topic; will be taken into consideration.

Chapter 2

Philosophy and Zarathushtra

In the beginning part of this chapter we will have a quick look at topic of Philosophy, and Zarathushtra's place in this field. Then, there will be a look at Zarathushtra's life and his message. Beforehand it is useful to mention some background information about the names that will be mentioned in different parts of this writing. First, the words "Zarathustra", "Zoroaster", "Zardosht" and "Zartosht" all refer to the same person 'Zarathushtra'. Different scholars, writers, and people have used these different names for referring to Zarathushtra.

Second, the book which contains Zarathushtra's teachings is called "The Gathas". In the following parts of this text there is a word called "Gathic", which refers to what is related to; the Gathas. For instance Gathic vision means the vision of the Gathas. "Zarathushtrian", "Zartoshti", "Zardoshti", "Parsi/ Parsee" -in India-, "Zarthoshty" and "Zoroastrian" all of them refer to a person who is a follower of Zarathushtra either counting him as prophet, philosopher, master or/ and teacher. Third, "The Avesta" is an ancient Zoroastrian literature, which also includes the Gathas; but except the Gathas none of its other parts is said by Zarathushtra.

Philosophy

2.1

According to Parkinson (1996, 1) the word 'Philosophy' has its roots in ancient Greek's language. The Greek word 'Philosophia' literally means 'Love of Knowledge' -philo means love and sophia means knowledge-. And for many of the Greeks, a philosopher was seeking almost any kind of knowledge.

In several songs in the Gathas, Zarathustra encourages loving wisdom; and this meets the concept that was described about philosophy. Zarathustra named God "Ahura Mazda", Ahura means Self-existing One, or Existing One; and Mazda signifies Wisdom. In addition, Zarathustra's God is also acknowledged as "Lord Wisdom". By taking these into consideration, alongside being a religious person, Zarathustra was, undoubtedly, the first philosopher that we know in history. (Abreu 2009, 55-56)

Ethics is the philosophical science accountable for the studies concerning what is, right and what is, wrong. The majority of philosophical researchers considers Socrates, Plato, and Aristotle as the first contributors to the concepts on ethics. But by considering Socrates's birth on 470 BC, Plato's birth on 428 BC, Aristotle's birth on 384 BC, almost 1305 years before Socrates, Plato, or Aristotle even born; Zarathushtra found that the human world on earth is categorized into two areas of righteous and wrongful. (Abreu 2009, 55)

According to Nasr & Aminrazavi (2007, 1) "In ancient times, however, Persia was known to the Occident also as the land where the sun of philosophy shone so brightly that Plotinus entered the Roman army with the hope of going to Persia to encounter its philosophers. Moreover, when what remained of the Platonic Academy was closed by the Byzantines, the philosophers residing there took refuge in Persia. As far as Zoroaster, the prophet of ancient Persia, is concerned, he was known in the ancient world not only as a prophet but also as a philosopher."

2.2

"But he [Zarathushtra] was the watcher in the night, who stood on the lonely peak facing the East and broke out singing the poems of light to the sleeping world when the sun came out on the brim of the horizon. He declared that the sun of truth is for all, that its light is to unite the far and the near. Such a message always arouses the antagonism of those, whose habits have become nocturnal, whose vested interest is in the darkness." (Tagore)

According to Zoroastrian tradition, Zarathushtra was born on 26 March 1767 BC. His mother's name was Dughdav, and she was well-known for her enlightened opinions and ideas. His father's name was Pourushaspa of the Spitama clan -an Iranian tribe-, and he used to raise cattle and he was well-known for his horses. Zarathushtra was inquisitive person, who was; thoroughgoing thinker. (Abreu 2009, 17)

After years of doing meditation, thinking, and observation in East side of Iran's high mountains; Zarathustra was 30 years old when he came across the most tremendous principle on which he established his timeless philosophy of existence. This existential philosophy is that "The aim of existence is to lead a happy life and the aim of life is to take part in the betterment of the world, where ever living being, humans, animals and plants live in peace and plenty". He exposed this principle and how to achieve it in the Gathas. (Khazai 2007, 38)

Zarathushtra's Worldview

2.2.1

Zarathustra's thought provoking book is called "The Gathas". It contains 17 songs, sang by Zarathustra. These 17 songs have come from Zarathustra's mouth almost 4000 years ago and they have reached to us unchanged. The Gathas is the core of Zarathustra's doctrine or existential philosophy and it is based completely on reason as well as wisdom. (Khazai 2007, 10-16)

The Gathas' language is one of the ancient Iranian languages, and it was spoken in the east of greater Iran. The language of the Gathas is relevant to the Sanskrit language, but several centuries older. Since 19th century, we know that the Gathas' language is not just the source of entire Iranian languages, but also for many European languages it is one of their sources. (Khazai 2007, 11-14)

In the Gathas two types of world, including material world -physical world- and intellectual world, are mentioned. One of these two worlds is made of material and another one is made of thought. Material and intellectual worlds are interrelated. The human being lives and moves in these two different worlds simultaneously. For instance human breaths, but s/he also thinks constantly. (Khazai 2007, 21)

Ritualistic is the least in the Gathic ethic. The only offering, which is required; is offering of good actions. Besides, teachings of the Gathas tell us that only through thoughts, words, and actions human prepares her/his afterlife destiny. Indeed, human's "daena" -spiritual double- turns to ugliness or beauty according to her/his deeds in life. (DuBreuil 1984)

In Zarathushtra's point of view world is constantly in movement, evolution, and progression and it is going towards perfection. There are forces that are creative, called 'spenta mainyu', and they are all the time refreshing and renewing this world. Spenta mainyu literally means progressive mind. Zarathushtra guides that for reaching a happy life and creating a happy world, women and men should coordinate their thoughts, words, and actions; with spenta mainyu -creative forces-. Human should seriously take responsibility for contributing in this creative process, and they should be a help to God on the way of evolution for moving the world towards perfection. (Khazai 2007, 26)

All cells and all organs live, and for that thanks to these two worlds' unity. As long as someone's body and mind are connected together and they work in harmony and unison, s/he can live happily and can lead a healthy as well as joyful life. On the other hand, disharmony between material and spiritual worlds brings illness, and a break between these two worlds means physical death. The material world is vulnerable and ephemeral, but the intellectual world -spiritual world- is eternal. Hence, when physical body ends, this does not mean that is the end of life. Life goes on in the spiritual world -world of thought- that is eternal. In the Gathas, Zarathushtra explains the principles that lead humans into a happy life in both physical as well as spiritual worlds. (Khazai 2007, 21-22)

God in Zarathushtra's Worldview

2.2.2

In his book Hyperspace, Machio Kaku expresses, he has found it helpful to carefully categorize meanings for the expression "God" in two distinguished groups. It is sometimes useful separating between the God of Order and the God of Miracles. When scientists apply the word God, what they usually mean is the God of Order. (Anoshiravani)

It can be precisely declared that Zoroastrianism stands on believing in a universal order, value of divine knowledge, sense of reason, and freedom of choice. In some opinions, Zarathushtra, in explaining his religious doctrine; he has almost reached what can be named 'scientific precision' in today's phrasing. (Anoshiravani)

Abreu (2009, 13) refers that the Gathic term "Vohumanah" which means the good mind, is the origin of all that is good and wise. Zarathushtra discovered, recognized, and attained God via his own good mind. Khazai (2007, 23) points out that Zarathushtra named God "Ahura Mazda". This name is translated by various authors as the super wisdom, the universal source of wisdom, the supper intellect, the great knower, the great knowledge, the essence of life and wisdom or the God of life and wisdom. One of the most considerable Zarathushtra's discoveries was to discover this God. The God that Zarathushtra discovered and taught about it, was not similar to previous gods that people knew. The previous gods that people knew were strong, cruel and retaliating phenomenon, who wanted blood of sacrificed innocent animals.

Zarathushtra discovered that God is wisdom endowed with every good quality like progress, creativity and love. Ahura Mazda the God that Zarathushtra discovered is progressive and has made a dynamic universe. And, in the universe that Ahura Mazda created; everything is progressing towards perfection. (Khazai 2007, 23)

Ahura Mazda owns six attributes, and these are pure abstractions. These attributes do not have individuality and they do not have a mythology. These are spiritual ideals and in the Gathas' system they have a fundamental role to play. These attributes are included of "Asha" or Righteousness, "Vohu manah" or Good Thought, "Khashatra" or Self-Dominance, "Armaiti" or

Serenity, "Haurvatat" or Evolution and perfection, "Ameretat" or Immortality. (Khazai 2007, 26-29)

Zarathushtra's Influence in Human Society

2.2.3

About 1700 BC, Zarathustra established the earliest fellowship for those seekers of wisdom; who, were searching for understanding existence phenomenon. He named that fellowship "Assembly of Magi". "Magi" which is a plural word, comes from the word "Maga" that is repeated many times in the Gathas; and it means high in wisdom or great. It refers to those people who are seeking throughout wisdom. Members of this assembly could speak about existence, happiness, life, serenity, death, love, deception, wickedness friendship, and separation; but, strictly on the basis of wisdom. Pupils of Zarathustra named him "manthran", which means the Teacher/ Master. (Khazai 2007, 31)

Zarathushtra's manner to teach is shown clearly through the Gathas' songs. His method is surprisingly modern. It can be said it is timeless. His approach is built on awakening the brain, stimulating the thought, and refreshing and widening one's perspective on life. His technique is founded on "asking questions and searching for the answers". Zarathushtra does not admit anything unless he figures it out with his wisdom. He questions everything again and again, and he never stops until he grabs the answer. He is aware that nothing should stay in darkness because darkness opens the doors widely to superstition and deception. (Khazai 2007, 33)

Greek philosophers continually used Zarathushtra's name as a symbol and representation of knowledge. But surprisingly, many of them guarded their own scientific or philosophical work under the fictitious cover of Zarathushtra's authority. Aristotle points out a very extreme date of 8500 years ago about Zarathustra's date of birth. On the other hand, there is a general belief that some great philosophers like Plato, and Pythagoras studied in Zarathushtra's school. (Khazai 2007, 37-39)

Jenny (2011, 240) indicates that "Classical texts, such as Pliny's Natural History, Porphyry's Life of Pythagoras, Clement of Alexandria's Stromata and Apuleius' Florida, which speak of Zoroaster as the instructor of the Greeks in philosophy, astrology, alchemy, theurgy and magic, appealed to early Renaissance clerics and scholars in their search for a more rounded picture of the created world and the sequence of historical progress than was provided by the Christian church of the time. During the Renaissance, these texts, studied in the original, became the sources of reference regarding the ancient world. Certain Christian scholars were greatly influenced by the Greek perception of Zoroaster as a figure of authority and wisdom, preceding the great philosopher, such as Pythagoras and Plato. Others perceived Zoroaster as a transforming magician, astronomer and alchemist. For some, the two facets were connected. This reinvented 'Zoroaster' was accorded authority as a humanist voice that addressed the dilemma of the age."

Georgius Gemistus -Giorgius Plethon-, who was influential and great Byzantine philosopher in the 14th and the 15th century; by the help of his Jewish master Eliaus began walking into the Zoroastrian philosophy. He tried to establish a universal religion being made of Zoroastrianism and Platonism. Plethon's ideas expanded among the European elite. It then grew inside the Platonic Academy of Florence. His ideas became the groundwork for the process, which reached to humanism in Europe at the time of the Renaissance. (Khazai 2007, 43)

Interest in Zarathushtra was reborn again from that period. However, everything required to be rediscovered such as the language that Zarathustra's thought was transcribed, but it was forgotten for almost 2000 years. It was in the 18th century that Anquetil Duperron, who was a French scholar, could translate the Zoroastrian texts called "the Avesta". But on the other hand, Avesta is not Zarathushtra's work. In fact, it is made of different texts; which were written centuries and even a thousand years before or after Zarathushtra. (Khazai 2007, 43)

It was in 1861 that Martin Haug, who was an intelligent philologist by splitting Zarathushtra's words -the Gathas- from other parts of the Avesta, could succeed translating them. Yet, we should know the fact that his translation had certain numbers of significant errors. Farther philological as well as historical research provided that the Gathas' 17 chapters, were exactly the words that Zarathustra told them from his own mouth almost 4000 years before. (Khazai 2007, 45)

The Gathas' Social, Environmental, and Organizational Aspects

2.3

In the following parts of this chapter we will have a glance at Zaratustra' taught related to three aspects in topic of Corporate Social Responsibility. As mentioned in introduction part, CSR and the Gathas, each of them includes a wide variety of aspects. Therefore, in this book only three aspects, which deal with Environment, Society, and Organization, will be taken into consideration. In this chapter, these aspects will be looked from Zarathushtra's point of view and the next chapter will focus on them from CSR's outlook.

"Hear the best with your ears and ponder with a bright mind. Then each man and woman, for his or her self, select either of the two. Awaken to this Doctrine of ours before the Great Event of Choice ushers in." The Gathas: Song 3.2 (Jafarey's translation, 1989)

As mentioned earlier, Zarathustra used the term "Ahura Mazda" for calling the only God and creator of the entire material and physical worlds. From a grammatical point of view, this term is both masculine and feminine. Ahura means the being/ the essence, which is the masculine part of the name; and Mazda means the super wisdom/ the origin of wisdom, which is the feminine part. This perfect grammatical construction for naming God, who is both feminine and masculine, does represent the stringent equality of women and men in Zoroastrian system. One of the bases that Zoroastrian system stands on it, is this stringent equality of human genders. (Khazai 2007, 22-23)

Abreu (2009, 56) indicates that from the Gathas' perspective, women and men should enjoy equal rights. In the Gathas, genders are considered equally and there is no gender discrimination. Khazai (2007, 40) refers that Paul du Breuil, who is a French specialist of Zarathushtra, indicates that "the Persian women enjoyed the unprecedented liberty through the whole Antiquity, thanks to Zarathushtra's reform".

Freedom of choice is another base of Zarathustra's teachings. Every woman and man can freely make a choice about her or his vision and way of life, either good or bad. Besides, this freedom of choice entitles every individual; either woman or man a responsible person for her or his own happiness or misery. On the other hand, we discussed that in the Gathas human beings are considered as creator's co-workers for bringing this world into a happier place for all living beings. In short human being has freedom of choice, to choose her/ his way of life and this makes her/ him responsible for two things, one is being responsible for her/ his own happiness and another one is being responsible for improving the imperfections of this world towards perfection. (Khazai 2007, 24-25)

In Zoroastrian terms, a person that wishes to make a good choice in order to live a happy life; needs to pick the wisdom that will lead her/him to the source of wisdom -Ahura Mazda-. Wisdom in Zoroastrian terms, is the power that brings people the ability for distinguishing between bad and good, injustice and justice, deception and righteousness, stagnation and progress, hatred and love, anxiety and serenity, sadness and joy, animosity and friendship, misery and prosperity. Bad signifies the forces that prevent people from reaching happiness, and good signifies the forces that drive them towards happiness. (Khazai 2007, 25)

As a result, in Zoroastrian term wisdom is considered better than any knowledge. If knowledge is not driven by wisdom, it is destructive. On the opposite, if knowledge is driven by wisdom; it guides towards happiness. The world as creature of Ahura Mazda is constantly in movement, evolution, and progression and going towards perfection. (Khazai 2007, 26)

As already mentioned the Gathas talks about creative forces called spenta mainyu -progressive mind-. All people, both women and men are guided to harmonize and coordinate their thoughts, their words, and their deeds; with spenta mainyu. Each individual is suggested doing so in order to reach a happy life for herself/ himself, and also in order to create a happy world. Human is guided to take responsibility for contributing in this creative process actively, and support Ahura Mazda on the way of evolution for moving the world towards perfection. (Khazai 2007, 26)

Zarathushtra continually complains about the cruelty and violence that he notices in the society. He directs people for choosing righteousness. But few numbers of human beings willfully make a choice to be evil. These people simply decline in exercising their good mind in order to choose good. Concerning human evil, we should know that is fundamentally a disordered condition. Human evil is a collapse of the moral faculty, but not an operating pursuing of the wrong. Zarathushtra realizes this in the Gathas –Song 3.3-. In this part of the Gathas Zarathustra contrasts the nature of bad and good people. He does not announce that a good person chooses virtuously, but the devil person chooses wickedly. But instead he announces that a good person chooses wisely, and the evil person does not. The source problem is failing in making moral choice. (Bailey)

"The twain spirits which appeared in the world of thought in the beginning were good and evil in thoughts, words and deeds. The wise will choose rightly (of the said two thoughts), but the unwise shall not do so and shall go astray." The Gathas: Song 3.3 (Azargoshasb's translation, 1980)

"I pray to Thee, O Mazda, with uplifted hands, and to thy Holy Spirit, first of all and hope that through truths and righteousness I would enjoy the light of wisdom and a clean conscience, thus bringing solace to the Soul of (Mother Earth) Creation." The Gathas: Song 1.1 (Azargoshasb's translation, 1980)

In Zarathustra's message the aim of life is, living in a joyful and happy existence on the earth and uniting with the 'world of thoughts' or spiritual world, which is linked to the physical world. It is important to know that in his message, this happiness does not consider only human beings, but quite the opposite. Human should take responsibility for bringing happy life for animals as well as plants that they flourish their whole lives. An individual can not drive a happy life in a miserable and gloomy environment or society. Zarathustra taught that for achieving this happiness the key is to establish a society that stands on the righteousness, prosperity and progress, and serenity. (Khazai 2007, 19-20)

Zarathushtra's Gathas does not describe God as the merchant who gives benefits to those people that gratify him. Rather, God is the source and the creator and designer of the universal order –Asha-. Universal order determines the reaction to each and every action and the consequence of each and every behavior and action. (Anoshiravani)

According to the Gathas, this consequence and reaction is totally independent from God's gratification or dissatisfaction. This kernel perception accomplishes a conversion in the focal point of control and human responsibility, without lowering creator's divine authority. In addition, this also makes human beings empowerment and motivates her/him to learn the laws of nature as well as attainment of divine knowledge. When human realizes the laws of nature and understands the system of consequences, s/he discontinues soothing God for remarkable grant and privilege. Instead, s/he starts thinking, speaking, and acting in a manner compatible with God's eternal and universal order, and accordingly s/he becomes righteous. (Anoshiravani)

Teachings of Zarathustra are eco-compatible. They announce that all things in nature are divine creations. Human should deeply respect and love everything in nature. Zarathustra's doctrine supports an increasingly ecological order in a very scientific manner. (Abreu 2009, 56)

Previous to all other spiritual guidance, Zoroaster denounced all kinds of human exploitation by another human; as well as all kinds of persecution of animals. One may refer to Plato, Scholia, and Pliny the Elder to find out about the Greek tradition concerning Zoroaster's vegetarianism. Appreciating life and respecting animal welfare recently has become Western conscience's new achievement, and for that thanks to admirable thinker such as Mahatma Gandhi and also Dr. Albert Schweitzer, but still thousands of years ago Zarathushtra preached it. (DuBreuil 1984)

"And whoever foils the wrongful by word, thought, or action, or if approached by a visitor, teaches him good things, advances in his convictions to the satisfaction of the Wise God." The Gathas: Song 6.2 (Jafarey's translation, 1989)

In this respect, from a Zoroastrian point of view the entire society, either as leaders, organizations, or an individual; all of them are requested for championing Truthfulness, and Righteousness, as well as other noticeable manifestations of goodness, but not for the rewards that they may get, or due to well things that will be reflected upon them. They are requested to do so just for the goodness sake, not for any other reason. Human has a duty to make choices and the ideal choice is the one which is parallel to bringing enlightenment and harmony. (Abreu 2009, 94)

In Gathic Model, people are reminded that they need to make choices in their daily life and they need to make the right ones. When it is about making a moral decision, people are expected to gain the ability to consider others' welfare, and to keep a distance from pure self-interest. Through choosing the path of righteousness, welfare, happiness, and harmony for all will be promoted. (Abreu 2009, 94)

Promoting serenity in organizations raises friendly and peaceful relations. By doing so arrival of violent expressions that can become a threat to wellbeing of organization can be avoided. Violent expressions from a managerial point of view are unwanted and undesirable conditions in the organization. And, by promoting serenity; these conditions will be decreased. (Abreu 2009, 103)

It can be understood from Gathic teachings that serenity boosts individual success as well as organizational prosperity. Besides, acting righteously produces progressive serenity. The Gathas also teaches that ethical leaders, who support righteousness in their thoughts, words, deeds, and consciences; they belong to growing serenity and they are awarded with wholeness as well as immortality. (Abreu 2009, 103-105)

From a Zoroastrian point of view, a Good Mind is the main element for supporting an ethical framework for organizations. When the mind is absorbed in Serenity –Aramaiti-, a Good Mind rises and in this state of mind it is easy to cultivate and propagate unlimited numbers of other ethical values in organizations, society and humans. This model is the guideline for establishing an ideal organization. (Abreu 2009, 99)

In management field, among all diversities of ethical thoughts; Zarathustra's teachings are gaining position. For this the reason is that historically, the earliest formal ethical document introduced to humankind is the Gathas. Each song in the Gathas raises the cultivation of values. And by studying the Gathas, it can be deduced that "The Theory of Values" had its earliest roots in Zarathustra' philosophical teachings. The original sources of the ethical values that human apply in daily life; can be found in the Gathas. (Abreu 2009, 41-48)

Zoroastrian ethical philosophy consists of the earliest historical formulation of virtues, values, and principles. This ethical philosophy can comfortably be applied to the modern management. The groundwork granted by good thoughts, words, and deeds -good thinking, communication, and actions- directs to the three secure pillars for the Quality Management. (Abreu 2009, 149)

In addition, the Gathas offers the tools which can be taken into use to establish a powerful foundation for Human Resource Management –HRM- in order to attain excellence. For example, the Gathic vision provides the possibility of approaching body, mind, and spirit of the organizations. This ethical thought boosts spiritual and material progress of the world, organizations, and people who are a part of them. (Abreu 2009, 129-130)

"Vohu – Khshathra" is used to formulate the Zoroastrian Theory for Human Resource Management. Vohu means good. And the meaning of Khshathra is settling in peace, ruling a settlement, indicating "power" for settling people in peace. Vohu-Khshathra stands for benevolent power, the chosen order, and good rule. It demonstrates the ideal government in both matter and spirit. Organization's excellence can be obtained only by good thinking, justice, and righteousness. (Abreu 2009, 129-130)

The good rule -Vohu-Khshathra- in HRM is a perfect organization's vision that welcomes both employees and employers, together, targeting the same goals; in a benevolent environment. The resounds of this thought is coming from an ancient time, but they are still fresh; and they are promoting both human progress and tolerance. In organizational policies, actions of the benevolence drive to ideal and perfect strategies for HRM; which successively contribute in making an ideal society. (Abreu 2009, 130)

HRM deals with people, and people are the most important and vital part of an organization. In this regard, Zoroastrian theory for HRM includes a potent humanistic base. Zoroastrian point of view recognizes human resources to be an organization's most essential force; technology and machines are just intermediate instruments that are between that force and approaching the organizational goals. This model involves a responsibility of social-cultural, for every company. (Abreu 2009, 130-131)

In recruiting process in Zoroastrian methodology for HRM, besides the candidates' technical capability; there is an important attention to their attitudes and values. The admission test should contain evaluating candidates' capacity for friendship, and their teamwork ability. In this model HRM shows the most important path that through it organizations advance and motivate their employees, for cultivating their behaviors and increased productivity to be company's assistant; for achieving its business objectives and its valued-founded goals. (Abreu 2009, 131-132)

Vohu – Khshathra promotes a very powerful collection of values, which feeds the culture of the organization. This set of values, is an expression of a good mind; which strongly emphasize teamwork, community, and serving other people. It supports that organization's employees are a piece of a family, and they are encouraged for taking care of each other and also taking care of customers. Besides, employees as a part of the family; are inspired to be a unit of the organization and they are permitted for participating in activities of the company. In an organization that operates like a community and it has a significant aim in spiritual levels, the employees of that organization discover a worthwhile work. In this way, employees recognize that they are assisting in the mission of this particular organization. This manner motivates employees' feeling of partnership with other staff, with the organization itself, and with society. (Abreu 2009, 132)

In this model, some vital aspects of the Zoroastrian notion of business are there; for providing relationships that result nurturing, caring, and cooperation. The community's work is considered valuable, but simultaneously it is expected that both employees and managers work hard. This hard-working effort is founded on the responsibility, which comes from being part of an organization that has significant goal. These ethical view's elements are parallel with the criteria that a superb organization is integrated by personnel, who are enthusiastic, anxious to point out their ideas, hardworking, and loyal to the organization. (Abreu 2009, 132)

Teachings of Zarathustra offer guidance to individuals to attain enlightenment and immortality without rejecting mental freedom, physical freedom, or freedom of choice. This attribute appreciates human rights' topic. In the Gathas there is no gender, race, color, or nationality discrimination. (Abreu 2009, 56)

Importance of Worldview Concerning Organizational Model

2.4

Dunphy and Stace (2002) indicate that if we see the universe as a machine, then we start establishing organizations that they stand on the machine metaphor. In this model employees are inside the machine, and managers are outside organization for controlling employees and everything inside. For making something with that machine or for something to be happening, managers need to push some particular buttons and so forth. This creates a kind of command and control model of management for an organization. (Bubna-Litic 2009, 44)

On the other hand, philosopher Alfred North Whitehead suggests an opposite point of view against mechanistic model, which is titled as organic view. According to Whitehead, the connection between thought and life is very strong. He suggests that "As we think, we live". The reason that for this view, 'organic' view is gained; is that the machine metaphor is displaced with the living organism. (Bubna-Litic 2009, 44 - 45)

Importance of Personality Concerning Social Responsibility

2.5

For an individual, believing in social responsibility's rightness is tied up to that person's personality; where attitudes and values and thinking patterns have an important role for playing in the way that s/he conducts and judges herself or himself. White (2004) presents Political Apathy Disorder –PAD- as a new personality disorder. In an easy to understand words, PAD reflects a failure for engaging in activity that is designed to reduce others' suffering. A person with PAD has moved to an apathy status, where s/he no longer cares about her/ his lack of motivation of helping others. Such a person lacks sufficient empathy and lacks compassion to push action on behalf of those people who are outside her/ his inner circle. (Crowther & Capaldi 2008, 223-224)

It is good to know that such apathy that has been explained can be cured. Now in here, a useful way is presented for increasing individuals' considerations for helping others. Some people only need to watch the news about a particular situation or to read about it, in order of becoming aware. But this is not the case for many people who need to experience the pain in the relatives' eyes or in the loved ones' eyes. One way to gain deeper knowledge about issues, implications and results of other people's need is socialization. Social conscience can be developed by the help of social awareness. When social conscience develops, it awakens both ethical behavior and moral in managerial decisions as well as actions. (Crowther & Capaldi 2008, 224)

Moral awareness is defined as "a person's recognition that his/her potential decision or action could affect the interest, welfare, or expectations of the self or the others in a fashion that may conflict with one or more ethical standards." When it comes to social conscience, we should remember; it is necessary that individuals pass from the status of just having conviction about something; to the status of taking an action that represents the will of social conscience. Academics that are contributed in educating tomorrow's managers, have the moral obligation for awakening a concern in their students to consider responsible practices; to help them increase their social awareness and their social conscience that will support the incidence of making ethical action and making moral decisions. In this arena academia hold a moral responsibility to both humanity and the planet. (Crowther & Capaldi 2008, 224-227)

Now, concerning what have been discussed; we look back at Zarathushtra's worldview. According to Khazai (2007, 22) Zarathustra named his doctrine 'Daena vanguhi' that means good conscience. He called his teaching 'Manthra', which means thought awakening words. Zarathustra's disciples gave him the title of The Teacher 'Manthran'. Manthran means the person who instructs thought awakening songs. Later on Zarathustra's disciples named his teachings the Gathas, which means the sublime songs.

Chapter 3

Corporate Social Responsibility –CSR-

The idea of CSR is not new. It can be traced back to thousands of years ago. According to BRASS (2004) "In ancient Mesopotamia, around 1700 BC, a king introduced a code in which builders, innkeepers or farmers were put to death if their negligence caused the death of others, or major inconveniences to local citizens." (Paetzold 2010, 3)

But in earlier history, it seems that acting responsible to the society by firms; started in the 18th century. According to Hond, F., de Bakker, F., & Neergaard, Peter (2007, 1) it was in that century when companies have taken steps into social responsible manners. They did so, through constructing houses and schools for the employees that were working for them, as well as for their employees' children.

Society in a large scale is convinced that modern businesses should not function just for ensuring long-term wealth for the organization, but they should have more duties and tasks for society. This was the general idea of CSR's concept. Society at large believes, businesses' stakeholders -including employees, consumers, the natural environment, government, and the community on a large scale- should be taken more seriously by the businesses. The approach of CSR concerns all organizations with different size, but people in the society take large companies to the center of attention; due to large companies' high-level of transparency. (Paetzold 2010, 3)

Lister (2011,16) suggests that "Corporate social responsibility is about the role of business in society, and societal expectations that companies will 'do good' by contributing skills, power, and resources to meet global sustainability goals. Nongovernmental organizations –NGOs-, governments, and industries around the globe have promoted CSR as a progressive, self-regulatory approach to achieving sustainable development."

For doing business in the 21th century, CSR has achieved an important place. No matter what someone feels about CSR, it is going to stay here. CSR has its importance for society as well as for business. In broad consideration, CSR is about building and maintaining social norms that bring economic markets to a more transparent and effectual level in serving societal interests. During decades, many different definitions for CSR have been presented through academics, councils, group and practitioners. (Beal 2014)

In the following paragraph author of this book, goes through an example about social responsibility objectives for a food-service company; in order to go towards the topic of social responsibility in a more perceivable way.

Social responsibility objectives for a food-service company can be objectives related to products' safety, honesty -for example not to offer or accept bribes- , staff's working condition, equal opportunity, business's sustainability, practicing ethical business, pay attention to over pollution and other environmental issues. A food-service company's social responsibility objectives emphasize the ethical aspects of that company's objectives. Many organizations consider a code of business ethics and social ethics to be good for their business. Besides, owning transparent social responsibility policies plays an important role, as progressively businesses will look for trading only with other businesses that they have such clear policies. (Cousins, Foskett & Pennington 2011, 41)

When corporate operation and societal values are changing very quickly, CSR can be an approach for matching these two parameters at once. Essentially ethical behaviour is a precondition for strategic CSR. Ethical behaviour of companies is the mirror image of their cultures. Company's ethical behaviour is a shared collection of values and guiding foundation, which is intensely rooted throughout its organization. (D'Amato, Henderson & Florence 2009, 6)

Concerning global poverty and climate change, the choice of 'to do nothing' is not viable anymore. Rather, it is about questioning. The question is what action will be taken by companies and also affirming that companies' decisions will bring long-term association on the planet earth as well as on profits. For more urgent local problems, it is also necessary to take an action. But often the science and evidence are partial. Therefore, rather than putting effort to establish one single CSR formula suitable for all different situations, it is important to know the 'principles' of CSR. (Wall 2008, 17)

There are existing opportunities for companies to be taken into use in order to establish shared value. It sometimes needs that companies make difficult decisions and also the solution might not always be obvious. But by the help of using a company's core competence in order to build value for society, there will be also existing opportunities to improve shareholder value. (Wall 2008, 46)

In answering the question of 'what to do' considering CSR in different companies, we do not have one single solution; and, challenges for each company and industry differ from one to another. However, depending on how companies make use of their core competences to establish shared value, they can establish competitive advantage; and also depending on that they will progressively define their relation to society and their corporations. Like any other decision making in business, in here also the challenge is outperforming the competition and innovating to establish new solutions to earlier intractable problems. In order to make that company should enhance its core competence to establish shared value. (Wall 2008, 46)

Until now in this writing, we see that both CSR and Zarathustra's message do not provide one single solution for what to do in all different cases. Just the opposite. They provide the groundwork and principles, which can guide for decision making concerning each unique case. In this regard, here we look back to Zarathustra's point of view; to see how his guidance can be used for recognizing the required ingredient to create CSR's formula. For this purpose, in below; we go through writings of two scholars Abreu, J and Bard, A.

Abreu (2009, 41) indicates that an organization, which is integrated by a group of people who have the capability to generate wealth, capability to respond to social needs, and capability to evaluate the dimensions of their productivity; is a profitable organization. By taking this into consideration, one company forms an area which includes human relations, and that area can directly contribute to the establishment of a fair society. In this approach one of the fundamental "Life's Primary Principles" rapidly shows to be as a model for managing a company. And that model which tells us how to manage a company is "ASHA". Asha means truth, order, and righteousness.

Asha is "As the Universal law of righteous precision, which means 'to do the right thing, at the right time, in the right place, and with the right means in order to obtain the right result'". This concept of Asha creates the direction for making successful actions in management field, and through that the right results coming from the right decisions can vitally influence on the durability of all kinds of organizations as well as society. Asha is like something loving benefit and constructive, not just for an individual's own self, but also for her/his fellow creatures and for God. Asha is constructive, unselfish precision, and beneficial for excellence. Hence, for high-level management case, Asha is the best instruction; and the reason is that Asha delivers a shared prosperity to an organization, as well as to members of that organization, to the environment, and to society. (Abreu 2009, 41-42)

From the Zarathustra's teachings point of view, Good Mind -Vohu manah- should be the groundwork for taking any action, whether it is individual, social, or organizational action. The three uprights of 'Good Thoughts', 'Good Words', and 'Good Deeds' for achieving prosperity and perfection, emerge from Good Mind. Good Mind functions its wisdom, results these three mentioned pillars, and offers advantages for the individual behind of an action as well as advantages for an organization where that individual works in there and the society. In organizational aspects, selection of staff and leaders should be based on a good mind in order to bring righteous outcomes. (Abreu 2009, 35-36)

Zarathustra, after studying the human condition gained his existentialist conclusions. He characterized them as Asha. Modern science after studying the universe from its micro and macro perspectives gained similar conclusions. Hence, it is safe to announce that Asha's validity is supported on both facades. The universe operates according to a law, and that law is Asha. But in addition Asha is the law that human should live according to it, in order to be harmonious and constructive. (Bard 1998)

Implementation of CSR for Organization and Business

3.1

CSR has many benefits for companies, which can motivate them to implement and develop CSR policy. One of those benefits is that through CSR policy, companies' reputation can be improved in the consumer market. When a company's good social reputation increases, it can influence the consumers' buying decision for buying that company's product. (Paetzold 2010, 8)

Another benefit is that when a company achieves a good CSR reputation, it is expected to be more beneficial for the company through its current workforce as well as its potential employees. The logic is, when there is a better working atmosphere in a company due to ethical commitment coming from applying CSR policies, its current employees are more satisfied and more willing to do a better job in the company and therefore company's productivity increases, which results more profitability. On the other hand, as that company offers a good working atmosphere to its current employees; it will achieve a good reputation in comparison to its competitors and therefore, potential employees will be more attracted by this company. (Paetzold 2010, 9)

Hond, de Bakker & Neergaard (2007, 86) has listed some benefits of CSR for companies from different sources, which are worthy to be mentioned in here. These benefits were suggested in two categories of internal and external. Below we will go through these two categories.

Internal benefits of CSR are including of benefits from recycling and re-using of materials and energy, development of new services or products, savings coming through safer working conditions, improved morale of staff, development of organizational skills as well as managerial skills, products with higher quality, competencies and processes' systematization and competencies and processes' documentation, improvement of stuff retention and staff recruitment, saving from cost reduction of electricity and raw materials and so forth, increase in environmental awareness. (Hond, de Bakker & Neergaard 2007, 86)

External benefits of CSR are including of maintaining good reputation and enhancing it, improvement of company's image, having access to markets that they have demand for CSR, reduction of social risks and environmental risks, increase of responsibility of supply chain management, improvement of community relations, increase of competitiveness, legitimacy in society, compliance with environmental regulation and social regulation, better contact with public authorities and better cooperation with them, goodwill from stakeholders, brand value increases, price of products increases. (Hond, de Bakker & Neergaard 2007, 86)

CSR's Environmental, Social, and Organizational Aspects

3.2

The following parts of this chapter, aim to focus more on Environmental, Social, and Organizational aspects of CSR. Besides, at the beginning of going through each aspect; there will be a stanza from the Gathas –Zarathushtra's word-. The logic behind, is to emphasize the common points among Zarathustra's worldview and CSR; related to environmental, social, and organizational aspects.

"The Soul of the Living World lamented to You: Why did You create me? Who fashioned me this way? I am oppressed by fury, rapine, outrage, and aggression. I have no one to rehabilitate me other than You. Lead me to true civilization." The Gathas: Song 2.1 (Jafarey's translation, 1989)

The answer to the question, why we human must care about nature and look after it; has two reasons. One reason is that the nature does look after us as humans. And, the second reason is that other creatures that are not human, they have also intrinsic value. In an economic mind, natural world of animals and plants does not have value in itself and it just exists just to be used by human beings. But the truth is that in the cosmos, we humans are not the only one that has value in itself. And, this truth has both practical and ethical consequences. (Bubna-Litic 2009, 60)

On CSR topic, environment term is concerned with both responsibilities and opportunities. Corporate responsibility about environment deals with issues such as pollution, ecological degradation, waste management, natural resources' sustainable management, and energy management. Besides, some of business opportunities related to environment in CSR are including of ethical investment, green marketing, eco-efficiency, ethical consumerism/ green consumerism. (Visser, Matten & Pohl 2010, 157)

Pollution can be described as the spread of undesired from industrial production's product that break down the nature's quality or social environment. This spread can be into water, air, and soil; but visual pollution, light pollution, noise pollution, and radioactivity pollution can also be differentiated. Pollution can bring harm to health of fauna, flora, and human, to such a size that results extinction. Through pollution, substances that often do not exist in the natural environment are appended in such quantity that disturbs the biosphere's balance. Allergies, cancer, and different kinds of asthma are only some of the things that pollution can cause. (Visser, Matten & Pohl 2010, 317)

Although pollution and humanity are sharing the same age, but it was mainly in the late 19th and 20th century that pollution reached a high attention as a problem. It was during 1960s that consequences of pollution on the biosphere and ecosystem walked into the center of attention. During the 19th century many, countries released Clean Air Acts as well as Hindrance Acts. And also from the second half of the 20th century there has been the development for specific legislation related to soil protection, water pollution, waste management, noise control, and other crashes on the environment. (Visser, Matten & Pohl 2010, 317-318)

What climate change refers to, the variation in global weather systems of the earth over time. Several things are causing climate change. Amongst others, changes in the orbit of the earth, changes in vegetation, volcanic activity, variable solar activity, disastrous events like meteor impacts, and effect of greenhouse gases cause climate change. (Visser, Matten & Pohl 2010, 68)

The term of climate change recently has been used for describing additional anthropogenic -which is caused by human- deference to the climate. As this relates to an average grow in temperature, it is also noted as global warming. Additional greenhouse gases that are released through activities like deforestation, power generation, and transport case anthropogenic climate change. (Visser, Matten & Pohl 2010, 69)

If global warming continues to rise, global sea level will increase. As many people are living in coastal area, and as we people have developed our society; depending on the current climate and also accessing cheap energy, therefore global warming's effects on human society are expanded. (Visser, Matten & Pohl 2010, 69)

"Those persons would enjoy that previous reward which has been promised. O Mazda, who perform actions through knowledge and pure thought; who attempt for the progress and development of the world; fulfill the God's desire and try for the progress of God's Will through truth and righteousness." The Gathas: Song 7.14 (Azargoshasb's translation, 1980)

The aim of social rights is to ensure a specific living standard for individuals without any discrimination. Social rights include right to social security, right to a satisfactory living standard -for instance, right to satisfactory housing, cloth, and food-, and right to health. However, social rights are closely connected to economic rights. (Binder, Eberhard & Lachmayer 2010, 12-13)

Economic rights include rights such as right to work, right to have favorable and fair working conditions, right to form and join trade unions, and the right to free choice of employment. For the social rights, economic rights are counted as required precondition. It is via economic rights' realization that people can establish the financial foundation for the joy of social rights. (Binder, Eberhard & Lachmayer 2010, 13)

Climate change and poverty are considered to be the real problems. These two problems are particularly difficult in industries like oil, mining, travel, and textile industry; because in those industries, solutions to environmental and social problems are not unhesitatingly available or easy to implement. There is an increasing political and social consensus that businesses - especially multinational corporations- should accept their shared responsibility towards those problems. (Wall 2008, 2)

"The Wise God, of one accord with Righteousness, prepared His thoughtprovoking message in response to the sweet plea made by the World, because with His doctrine, He is the promoter for those who wish to be protected. He asked: Good Mind, do you know any person who can help the mortals?

Yes I do. There is only one person who has listened to our teachings. He is Zarathushtra Spitama. Wise One, he is prepared to proclaim the message through his Songs for the sake of Righteousness. Grant him sweetness of speech." The Gathas: Song 2.7 & 8 (Jafarey's translation, 1989)

Goldman, A (2006, 702) indicates that the culture of an organization develops during the time and it turns into a strong force for forming people's behaviour in that organization, as well as forming the behaviour of those who come as newcomers. Through two ways one organization can assist in having dysfunctional behaviour among its people. One way is that organization builds a social condition which supports violence by creating aggressive tendencies. The second way is that organization decreases limitations against violent performances.

Workplace deviance, aggression, theft, dishonesty, violence, and sabotage are some examples of dysfunctional behaviours. Scholars who work on the topic of dysfunctional work behavior, mostly they have concentrated on the particular individual-level behaviours. Most of them tend to reject or minimize the designation of organizational factors in influencing dysfunctional behaviours. (Goldman, A 2006, 699)

But on the other hand, it seems pretty likely that organizations also have an important role concerning dysfunctional behaviours. For taking this more into consideration, in here four points are mentioned that can make important of the organizations' role more understandable. Firstly, organizations provide a setting for people and it is in there, where individuals may show dysfunctional behavior. Secondly, is that an individual consumes most of the hours that s/he is awake at the working place, where again s/he can expose dysfunctional behaviour. Thirdly, it is an organization that arranges people that toward them; an individual may recognize it easier to expose dysfunctional behaviour, in comparing with her/ his family members that s/he loves them. And fourthly, work setting arranges all sorts of stimulus that could stimulate individuals, who have a high tendency for displaying dysfunctional behaviour. (Goldman, A 2006, 701)

Perhaps leaders are the mightiest determinant of organization culture and most likely they play a major role related to that. For instance, if a leader takes profits into consideration before anything else, if s/he does not have any respects for other people' s right, if s/he is known to be untruthful, all of these signals will likely be recognized by other people in the organization and will lead to dysfunctional culture in that particular organization. As dysfunctional behaviours, especially violence can cause damage or much cost to an organization, therefore organizations should be deeply concerned in preventing such behaviours at the workplace. Therefore, with respect to all that has been explained, values of a leader are 'taught' to other people of the organization and shape their behaviour. (Goldman, A 2006, 699,704)

CSR's Common Practices

3.3

In below, some common socially responsible practices in business are listed; which are adopted from Kotler & Lee (2005, 209-210).

- Designing facilities in order to meet or exceed safety and environmental guidelines and suggestions. For instance designing facilities for improving energy conservation.

- Improvements in developing a process that may involve practices like removing usage of hazardous waste materials, removing usage of particular oils in deep-fat frying, decreasing the amount of chemicals to be used for growing crops.

- Stopping product offerings, which are not illegal, but they are harmful.

- Choosing, supporting and rewarding those suppliers that are more willing to accept and maintain practices, which are environmentally sustainable.

- Selecting materials for packaging and manufacturing, which are in the highest level of being environmentally friendly, considering goals for waste reduction. Using resources that are renewable, and withdrawal of toxic emissions for packaging and manufacturing.

- Giving full disclosure about materials of the product and their origins as well as their potential hazards, and even offering extra helpful information related to the product.

- Improving programs for supporting the wellbeing of employees, like exercise facilities at the workplace.

- Tracking, measuring, and reporting; about accountable targets and actions, including both bad and good news.

- Creating instructions concerning to marketing to children, in order to assure suitable distribution channels and responsible communications. For instance, not to sell products online to underage children.

- Offering raised access for people with disabilities through using technology. For example, different print formats and mechanism with voice recognition.

- Securing the privacy of customers' information.

- Making decisions concerning outsourcing, retail locations, and factory; with considering these decisions' economic impact on communities.

Chapter 4

Short Story: The Magus and the King

Once upon a time there was a powerful king ruling a big territory. From morning to evening he was thinking and planning with his minister how to enlarge his kingdom. Inside his domain many people were struggling with daily hardship, and the king was not bothering himself about them; as he had a bigger objective to think.

The only thing that he was worrying was the size of his territory, and the number of success still left to be obtained. Meanwhile, there were always some moments in the king's mind that he was asking himself whether he is happy or not? Most of the time his answer was, "No, I am not yet, but I will be one day when I have bigger land and greater tributary under my rule."

Years used to come and go, and the king was just busy with his routine kingly life that one day he heard one Magus –Maga, who is high in wisdom- has walked to his kingdom; as a traveler. The king heard from his minister that the wise man has told to people about a lake of elixir for strengthening the body and mind, which increases happiness in life.

The king was amazed to hear about him, and wanted the stranger Magus to his palace. The king ordered him, "Stop telling your knowledge about the elixir to others and take me to the lake."

Magus started advising him that this way to go is not an easy one. It needs patience, not only about time; but also against being away from the king's comfortable palace on a long way adventure.

The king scowled and replied, "I am the greatest and I am not afraid of anything on the earth."

In the end the wise man's final request from the king was, "On the way to the lake of the elixir, which is not a short journey; you must put away all of your prejudice, proudness and selfishness. And, every day and night; you ought to listens to my speeches and try to find out lessen and motto out of them."

King scoffed clearly and accepted the deal for being humble and promised to try to think that although he is a king, but it does not mean he knows the best.

Soon journey started. For the king, the first two days were the most annoying part of it; as he was spending time with a Magus and trying to listen and understand his boring words and stories. There were some moments when king used to ask himself, "Did I make a correct decision of being along with a boring man, who knows a way to a lake of elixir that brings joyful life? His meaning of life might be as boring life as himself!"

But after few days slowly king was becoming interested in the Magus's speeches. With going through days, the time had come that after each speech king was asking for a break to go and think deeply in peace; about the ethics and motto that he learned from it.

Weeks passed one after one, and the king was just excited to listen and learn from the wise man; as these days he could watch the Magus's speech, not from his kingly and luxury position; but from his country people's eyes.

Every day was ending more interesting than previous one. Though their journey was getting shorter, but the king was losing his interest about the destination. Instead, he was becoming carrying about his kingdom and even more caring about his poor inhabitant in there.

One day when the Magus woke up to wake the king up for continuing their journey, he saw that the king is sitting under a cedar tree and he is gazing at the sky. He was thinking deeply, in silence. Peacefulness very clearly was showing up from the king's face.

The Magus started walking towards the king, to sit next to him. But suddenly the king stood up, and walked through him. He hugged the Magus and asked, "Let's forget about the lake of elixir and go back to my country. I want to be with my people".

The wise man rejected the king's request at first and replied, "You did not yet see the lake and you did not get the elixir".

The king replied, "Instead of finding the lake of elixir for bringing happiness, somewhere out there; I have found it inside me among other people."

The Magus smiled and said, "You found the better one".

On the way back home the king was asked by the Magus, "What you approached about the meaning of life and joy inside yourself that you think you do not need to find it from the lake anymore?"

The king replied, "For years I have been only busy with my goals and ambitions for trying harder and harder to get them that I had totally forgotten about everything else around me. I had forgotten about others and their life in my territory. I needed a break. I needed to live differently for some time to realize that happiness and life could have been always with me, but I did not know how. The elixir was inside your words and your teachings. I spent my life for getting stronger and gaining more power, and you spent your life in finding the reasons behind life's struggles. I started to drink another elixir when I started to listen to you and I learned humbly and delightfully. People around me are that happiness, which has not yet been discovered by me. Instead of the greediness for having new lands, I should have paid attention to help people to bring them happier and easier life; but I have brought them hunger and sadness. When they have the love of me in their hearts, I have the joy in me, which is influenced from hundreds of thousands of pleased people. And this is the real meaning of happiness in my life. Not a short life to be ended finally, but a long lasting life; as, a good memory about my kindness will be always told by next generations after generations. This is my true long lasting life."

References

Printed Sources:

Abreu, J. 2009. Seven Fires and Three Pillars of Ethical Management : The Zoroastrian Model for Good Business. Mexico.

Beal, B. 2014. Corporate Social Responsibility: definition, core issues, and recent developments. California: SAGE Publications, Inc.

Binder, C., Eberhard, H. & Lachmayer, K. 2010. Corporate Social Responsibility and Social Rights : Proceedings of the 5th Vienna Workshop on International Constitutional Law. Vienna: facultas.wuv.

Bubna-Litic, D. 2009. Spirituality and Corporate Social Responsibility : Interpenetrating Worlds. GBR: Ashgate Publishing Group.

Cousins, J. Foskett, D. & Pennington, A. 2011. Food and Beverage Management : For the hospitality, tourism and event industries. Third edition. Oxford : Goodfellow Publishers Ltd.

Crowther, D. & Capaldi, N. 2008. Ashgate Research Companion to Corporate Social Responsibility. Abingdon: Ashgate Publishing Group.

D'Amato, A. Henderson, S. & Florence, S. 2009. Corporate Social Responsibility and Sustainable Business : A Guide to Leadership Tasks and Functions. Greensboro: Center for Creative Leadership.

Goldman, A. 2006. Dysfunctional Leadership and Organizations. Bradford: Emerald Group Publishing Ltd.

Hond, F., de Bakker, F. & Neergaard, P. 2007. Managing Corporate Social Responsibility in Action : Talking, Doing and

Measuring. Abingdon: Ashgate Publishing Group.

Jenny, R. 2011. Zoroastrianism : An Introduction. London: I.B. Tauris

Jensen, R. 1999. The Dream Society : How the Coming Shift from Information to Imagination Will Transform Your Business. New York: McGraw-Hill.

Khazai, Kh. 2007. The Gathas : The Sublime Book of Zarathustra. Brussels : European Centre for Zoroastrian Studies.

Kotler, Ph. & Lee, N. 2005. Corporate Social Responsibility : Doing the Most Good for Your Company and Your Cause. USA : John Wiley and Sons, Inc.

Lister, J. 2011. Corporate Social Responsibility and the State. Vancouver: UBC Press.

Nasr, S.H., and Aminrazavi, Mehdi. 2007. Anthology of Philosophyin Persia, Volume 1 : From Zoroaster to Umar Khayyam. London, I.B. Tauris.

Paetzold, K. 2010. Corporate Social Responsibility (CSR) : An International Marketing Approach. Hamburg: Diplomica Verlag.

Paine, L. S. 1994. Managing for organizational integrity. Harvard Business Review.

Parkinson, G.H.R., ed. 1996. Encyclopedia of Philosophy. Florence, KY: Routledge.

Visser, W., Matten, D. & Pohl, M. 2010. A-Z of Corporate Social Responsibility. 2nd Edition. NJ: John Wiley & Sons.

Wall, C. 2008. Buried Treasure : Discovering and Implementing the Value of Corporate Social Responsibility. Sheffield: Greenleaf Publishing.

Electronic Sources:

Anoushiravani, A. Psychology of the Gathas;A Psycho-historical view of teachings of Zarathushtra. <http://www.gatha.org/index.php?option=com_content&id=264&Itemid=69&lang=en> (Accessed 16 March 2015).

Azargoshasb, F. 1980. Translation of Gathas : The holy Songs of Zarathushtra. <http://www.zarathushtra.com/z/gatha/az/The%20Gathas%20-%20FAZ.pdf> (Accessed 8 Sep 2015).

Bailey, A. Zarathushtrian Theodicy. < http://www.cais-soas.com/CAIS/Religions/iranian/Zarathushtrian/z_theodicy.htm > (Accessed 16 March 2015).

Bard, A. 1998. Zoroastrianism in the 21st Century – Preparing Ourselves for Mass Conversion. <http://www.zoroastrian.org.uk/vohuman/Article/Zoroastrianism%2 (Accessed 7 March 2015).

DuBreuil, P. 1984. New Scope on some Aspects of Zoroasrtrian History and Philosophy. <http://www.zoroastrian.org.uk/vohuman/Article/New%20Scope%2 (Accessed 7 March 2015).

Jafarey, A. 1989. The Gathas, Our Guide : the thought-provoking divine songs of Zarathushtra. California : Ushta Publication. <http://www.zarathushtra.com/z/gatha/The%20Gathas%20-%20AAJ.pdf> (Accessed 8 Sep 2015)

Osho. 1987. Zarathustra: A God That Can Dance : Commentaries on Friedrich Nietzsche's Thus Spoke Zarathustra. <http://www.oshorajneesh.com/download/osho-books/western_mystics/Zarathustra_A_God_That_Can_Dance.pdf> (Accessed 14 April 2015).

Tagore, R. The Divine Songs of Zarathushtra.

<http://www.zoroastrian.org.uk/vohuman/Article/The%20Divine%2
(Accessed 21 August 2015).